ESSENTIAL TRUTHS OF ALCOHOLISM

Practical Ways To Stop Drinking And Overcome Alcohol Addiction

Dr. Jose Pearson

Although the author and publisher have made every effort to ensure that the information in this book was correct at press time, the author and publisher do not assume and hereby disclaim any liability to any party for any loss, damage, or disruption caused by errors or omissions, whether such errors or omissions result from negligence, accident or any other cause. This publication is solely for personal growth and is sold with the understanding that neither the author nor publisher is engaged in presenting professional advice.

TABLE OF CONTENT

INTRODUCTION

Addiction is a condition that affects your mind and behavior. When you are addicted to a substance, you cannot resist the urge to use or consume it, no matter how serious the harm it may cause. The sooner you get help for addiction, the more likely you are to avoid the most serious consequences. The development of addiction is associated with several hereditary and environmental risk factors that differ in different population groups.

Hereditary and environmental risk factors each account for approximately half of the risk of existing addiction. In fact, exposure to sufficiently high levels of the substance over a long period of time (eg weeks-months) can lead to addiction in individuals with a fairly low hereditary risk. Research shows that youth abuse or exposure to violent crime has been positively associated with mood or anxiety complaints and the risk of substance abuse.

Addiction is quite easy to confirm because you can directly observe in yourself the repeated desire for goods and the resulting suffering. Ending addiction means fully understanding the addiction, which means staying with the addiction and fully controlling it. However, when someone suffers from addiction, they always want to be mentally free from the addiction, but this prevents them from observing and understanding.

Can you identify this tendency in yourself? Can you let go of all your desires and just stay with the problem and not run away from it? While it may be tempting to try some addictive strain for the first time, it's all too easy for the effects to go south, especially with alcohol or drug addiction. People develop tolerance when they abuse substances consistently over time. This means that larger amounts of drugs or alcohol are needed to achieve the desired goods, increasing the addictive nature.

Long-term alcohol abuse can lead to a dangerous cycle of addiction, where people must continue to use drugs or alcohol to avoid unpleasant withdrawal symptoms. By the time people realize they have a problem, drugs or alcohol may have already taken control, forcing addicts to prioritize drug abuse over anything else that was previously important in their lives. No one ever intends to become an addict. There are many reasons why someone tries a substance or behavior. Others are driven by curiosity and peer pressure, while others are looking for a way to relieve stress.

Children who grow up in environments where drugs and alcohol are present have a lower risk of developing a substance use disorder (SUD). Substance abuse affects many parts of the body, but it affects the brain the most. When a person uses alcohol or other addictive substances, the brain produces large amounts of dopamine; it triggers the price system of the brain.

After repeated alcohol consumption, the brain cannot produce normal amounts of dopamine on its own. This means that addicts may have difficulties finding pleasure in pleasurable exercise, such as spending time with friends or family, when they are not under the influence of alcohol. If you, a friend or family member is struggling with addiction, it is important to seek treatment as soon as time permits. Too often people try to heal themselves, but this can be tricky and sometimes dangerous.

Adverse childhood experiences (ACEs) are intermediate types of childhood maltreatment and home dysfunction. Studies of adverse childhood experiences conducted by the Centers for Disease Control and Prevention have shown a strong association between ACEs and a range of health, social and behavioral problems, including substance use complaints, throughout life.

A study of 900 court participants, including abused children, found that a large number developed some form of addiction during childhood or adulthood. This road to addiction, which opens with painful childhood encounters, can be avoided by adjusting natural variables throughout a person's life and having access to professional help. Family conflicts are also the reason why a person becomes addicted to alcohol or other substances. The devastating effects of addiction have a major impact on families.

To accommodate the habitual behavior of a friend or family member, families tend to keep secrets, look for scapegoats, and engage in regrettable behaviors such as denial, guilt, or distraction. So families need help doing their part to spot and treat addictive behaviors and build healthy boundaries and relationships. Researchers have also identified a number of social, spiritual, hereditary and miscellaneous elements that make some individuals more vulnerable to addiction than others.

In all cases, it is important to understand that no one chooses to be an addict. Two people can start using alcohol or other substances in the same way, with one person's use developing into a substance abuse disorder while the other has no symptoms. Remember that addicts cannot always use alcohol or other habitual drugs without jeopardizing their well-being. Their psyches have been altered so that they can be brought back into balance through rehabilitation, but the balance remains permanently weakened against constant use.

No single variable can predict the likelihood that a person will become addicted to an activity. A combination of different factors influences addiction. The more risk factors a person has, the greater the chance that such an activity will lead to addiction. For example:

Biology

Traits that people are born with account for about half of a person's risk of addiction. Gender, ethnicity and other mental health issues can also affect the risk of addiction.

Environment

An individual's current situation encompasses a wide range of influences, from loved ones to financial status and quality of life. Factors such as peer pressure, physical and sexual abuse, early exposure to drugs, stress and parental guidance can greatly influence a person's habits and addiction.

Development

Hereditary and natural factors are related to the risk of addiction, which affects the basic stages of human development. Although drinking alcohol at any stage of life can be addictive, it is more likely to develop into addiction than before drinking. This is particularly risky for young people because the areas of their brain that control direction, judgment and decision-making can be particularly vulnerable to risky behavior. You should understand that addiction cannot be overcome by accident.

It involves a moderate and complex cycle that occurs in an area of the brain known as the "reward center"—the very place that controls and maintains ordinary rewards essential to our reality, such as food and sex. To do this, the addict seeks alcohol and various vices, as if these substances are necessary for our survival. This is also the reason why people suffering from alcohol addiction put the search for alcohol before almost all other needs.

CHAPTER 1
SOCIETAL VIEWS

Alcohol itself is a substance that was once considered "God's good creature" by none other than Puritan preacher Cotton Mather, who considered alcohol a benign and healthy substance that should be consumed regularly by everyone, including children and pregnant women. Of course, the public sometimes had a radically different understanding of alcohol.

For example, at the end of the 19th century, alcohol in general, but also rum in particular, was perceived as an essentially bad substance. "Demon Rum" was believed by some to be highly and instantly addictive to anyone who foolishly chose to drink it, and was therefore believed to be a substance that should be actively avoided by all sane people. In later years, writers and supporters of Alcoholics Anonymous adopted the idea of alcohol as an irresistible substance for some people, for whom abstinence was the only salvation or relief.

(This belief in abstinence and abstinence among alcoholics is now supported by extensive research.) It is instructive and often helpful to learn about the beliefs and practices of people in the past. This historical overview examines the various views of alcohol, alcoholism and alcoholism, and alcoholics throughout history, beginning with medieval Europe and emphasizing alcohol consumption and abuse from colonial times to the present in the United States.

Attitudes towards alcoholics and alcoholics have also changed almost cyclically over time, and this introduction addresses society's changing views of alcoholics and attitudes toward their family members and co-workers. For example, an alcoholic at various times was considered morally degenerate, sick, weak, bad, suffering from an uncontrollable disease, etc. In today's society, many people consider alcohol addiction a disease, but there are still those who consider alcoholism a moral weakness.

There are also different views of society towards the family members of the alcoholic (especially the spouse). For example, the wives of drunken men at various times in history have been seen as tragic victims, people involved in the problem, or even people who somehow "drove" an alcoholic to drink. Attitudes, in general, were even more unfavorable to female alcoholics, who were seen as weak, lazy, bad, bad mothers, or, much less often, just people who needed help with their addiction.

This introduction discusses the changing attitudes towards female alcoholics and alcoholics over time. When looking at the past, it is important to consider society's views on alcohol at the time, not to overshadow modern views of the pilgrims who landed on Plymouth Rock, Victorian men and women, and other historical cultures or groups. If you know the opinions of the people of that time and their motives, their behavior is often much more understandable. In addition, the introduction has a separate section on the treatment of alcohol abusers throughout the ages, and this ranged from alcoholic bleeding (a remedy for many diseases in the 18th century) to drinking syrup or other extremely harmful substances. vomiting to counseling and social support and other resources.

Throughout history, some people abused alcohol, while others became addicted to it. Like attitudes toward those with substance abuse and addiction problems, attitudes toward people who abuse or depend on alcohol appear to have changed cyclically throughout history. Sometimes the alcoholic is seen favorably, especially when young, while the alcoholic can be seen as a victim of their culture or sometimes of alcohol itself.

From this point of view, it was believed that people are led to care by others who are more educated. Alternatively, alcoholics at various points in history were considered to have such a severe character or personality defect that they will never accept treatment and thus there is no way to help them because failure is inevitable.

In extreme cases, the alcoholic was seen as someone who really chooses to be bad, and sometimes as someone who should be removed from the pleasant people of society or imprisoned. One of the common denominators of these different points of view is that the alcoholic is either unable or unwilling to choose treatment for recovery.

Of course, alcoholism is not a positive trait for anyone, but it is important to understand that there are factors that put some people at risk for alcohol addiction, such as genetics and environmental factors (parents and/or peers who drink a lot). There are also protective factors that remove people from alcohol abuse and dependence (eg non-drinking parents and peers). At the same time, there are treatments that can help alcoholics. Another opinion about alcoholics or alcoholics is that the person is a free thinker who manifests an individual spirit.

People who have this point of view can see excessive drinking in some people, like the stereotypical drunken writer or artist, or the macho guy who really knows how to keep his alcohol good. In reality, the ability of heavy drinkers to drink more than others is due to the development of alcohol tolerance, and not to some secret knowledge acquired by the individual.

At various times in the history of the United States, alcohol itself was considered either good or bad. If it was good, it was perceived as a safe and healthy drink and pain. When it was bad, it was thought to be as addictive as heroin is known times today. According to this underlying view, no one was exempt from addiction. The belief that alcohol itself is extremely dangerous to everyone helps explain why this substance was completely banned during the Prohibition years. Others believed that not everyone is predisposed to alcohol, but that some people were inexplicably drawn to alcohol and eventually and inevitably became addicted.

According to this belief, the addiction was triggered by the first drink of alcohol. For such people, it resulted in a ruined life if they could not overcome their addiction with help. Social views of the non-alcoholic spouse or partner of an alcoholic have changed over time. In the early 20th century, women were often seen as innocent victims of drunken men.

This attitude changed in the 1950s and later when professional articles began to appear asking whether the problems of the male alcoholic were at least partly due to marital disorders. Women with alcoholic husbands were advised to look for the root cause of the problem within themselves. Lori Rotskoff said in her book Love on the Rocks: "This view was prevalent among mental health professionals in the late 190s and early 1950s, especially among those trained in psychoanalytic theory, which became increasingly popular during that period. "

Rotskoff also added that "psychiatric social workers considered the woman's behavior a sign of neurosis that existed before the partner's alcoholism began." Terms such as enabling have been developed to refer to certain behaviors that allow the alcohol behavior to continue. The prevailing belief (and still held by many people) was that when the enabling is over, the alcoholic must face his problem (usually seen as a male problem) and gain understanding and a desire to seek treatment.

Although spouses and family members are out of the picture, the alcoholic must admit to having a problem and seek treatment for it. Female partners of alcoholics were encouraged not to view themselves as victims but to learn to deal with their husband's problems by joining self-help groups such as Al-Anon and sending their teenage children to Alateen (Alcoholics Anonymous sister groups).

However, in many ways, non-alcoholic spouses were seen as part of the problem rather than the solution. Despite working to avoid enabling their husband or partner and faithfully attending Al-Anon meetings and receiving therapy, many women often find that their husband's alcoholic behavior continues anyway. Some women have concluded that they may not be trying hard enough, thinking that somehow they are still "getting" their male partners to drink.

CHAPTER 2
ACCEPTANCE

When you feel like this, it's so hard to get the inspiration, clarity, or energy to do anything to move forward. When we fight against reality, our actions make it difficult to adjust to the situation and our feelings. It doesn't go away either, because what you resist persists. Alcoholism or alcohol addiction does not only harm the consumer. Companions and offspring of alcoholics may encounter family savagery; children may experience physical and sexual abuse and neglect.

Women who drink during pregnancy risk harming their babies. Family members, friends, and strangers can be injured or killed in alcohol-related accidents and assaults. Once you understand the importance of coming to terms with your alcohol addiction, it's pretty important to seek help if you haven't already. There are various treatments available to help you recover from addiction. Your first step should be to talk to your primary care physician. The person can give you a referral and decide if the drug is an option for you. In addition to prescriptions, there are treatments to help you stop or reduce drinking, such as psychosocial therapy or stimulant medication.

Because solid family support increases an individual's chances of staying sober, treatment often includes marriage and family counseling. An alcoholic probably doesn't behave the way you expect him to. He can be knowledgeable and helpful. He may be a successful person or in an influential position. His wealth may make people overlook his drinking. He may also try to plead ignorance.

He might think, "I have a great job, I pay my bills, and I have lots of partners; that way I'm not addicted," or he might rationalize things like, "I only drink expensive wine," or "I haven't lost everything because drinking."

and have had no accidents." Many people believe they can fix the problem themselves, but that rarely works. Find someone to talk to. Unfortunately, overcoming addiction is not a one-day journey. Giving up alcohol is probably the hardest thing you or your partner will ever do. This is all but a sign of shortcomings if you want a ready guide or expert help.

A large number of people who are trying to nip alcoholism in the bud need professional help or a treatment program. Although alcoholics are constantly addicted to cravings, many find that their lives are improved after abstinence. They prefer not to think about going back to drinking, even if is sober. There are also many non-drinkers who try to drink lightly after collecting and conclude that life is better without drinking.

The correct answer to any recovering alcoholic who is considering a return to controlled drinking is to "remember your luck". This is sometimes called an "attitude of gratitude" and can be an effective antidote to faulty reasoning.

Types Of Acceptance

Acceptance Of Addiction And Reality

When it comes to alcohol use disorder (AUD) or substance use disorder (SUD), many people live in willful ignorance. It can include the person with the problem as well as family, partners, and co-workers and this is only the tip of the iceberg. For the person suffering from addiction, addiction often began as a way to withdraw from the real world. Usually, what starts as a habit of providing help becomes an important but wasteful method of escaping the real world.

This can be due to family or business-related pressures, as well as close pain caused by negative past experiences. When relief comes with the first drink, worries or problems also seem to disappear. Anyone who has faced a painful injury, nervousness, melancholy, rage, or any other uncomfortable and awkward feeling can attest that this brief escape is most welcome.

 Days become weeks, weeks become months and months become years almost in an instant what was a way to get better changed enough to live. Many are left asking themselves "how did I get here?". When addiction occurs, what used to be a way to feel better is expected to win the day or feel typical in some way. Anyone addicted to alcohol or other substances knows this well. It usually takes more of this substance to produce an underlying "high" or abnormality.

For some, this first impression of relief is the substance that was never found in the future. Either way, anyone with AUD or SUD continues to seek relief from the destruction of body, brain and soul. This often happens when the negation of the antonym of acceptance begins. When faced with the suggestion of consuming alcohol to ease this slide, the addict is completely out of touch with the real world.

Despite the unfortunate results many face from their habit, they continually deny that alcohol is a problem. Not only do they deny it to well-meaning friends and family who try to help, but they are also willfully ignorant, and this denial can be deadly. This denial can be deep, and the interesting part is that despite repeated difficulties due to drinking or alcoholism, the denial often persists.

Man has not only been deliberately ignorant for a long time, but it is terrifying to face reality. Chances that you don't have the chance to depend on alcohol and use it, you just have to deal with it a lot. This is where acceptance is crucial. Acceptance can begin with realizing and acknowledging that you may not fully understand the situation surrounding drinking or alcoholism. If you do it first, a small step of acceptance can pave the way to recovery and freedom. This acknowledgment that alcohol or some other substance has taken over his life is the first part of acceptance. Accept that alcohol is responsible, not the person themselves. This step can be difficult for some because it means accepting the fact that the substance that relied on so heavily for pain and anxiety is no longer working.

Self-Acceptance

When you recognize that you have AUD or SUD (or even both), you can begin to examine how you got there and what you need to do. This is one reason why it is important to choose an addiction treatment focus using evidence-based treatments and careful consideration. Experts agree and recognize that addressing all emotional well-being issues and different issues simultaneously is essential for sustained recovery. This is where self-acceptance comes in.

Addiction problems and emotional well-being follow signs of shame. It is really hard for some to admit that they have these problems. Regardless, self-acceptance is essential to recovery and peace of mind. Accepting yourself means accepting all aspects of yourself. The good and pleasant parts and the weaker and limited parts. Self-acceptance begins in childhood. To the extent that our parents or guardians have accepted us, we are able to accept ourselves.

Unfortunately, the acceptance of parents or guardians depends a lot on our behavior as children, not on who we really are. Some children are more adventurous, rebellious, independent and "hard to control". Then we begin to see many aspects of ourselves as negative, which leads to us not accepting who we really are. This unresolved pain and rejection from childhood can also lead you to turn to alcohol or drugs to "get better." This can be especially true when dealing with drug use is modeled at home. In contrast, it is important to turn to detoxification treatments that consider individualized, holistic and evidence-based treatment. A key place to start is to use both collection and individual care to address these blocks. Changing thoughts, like changing behavior and interacting with others, is important for self-acceptance. Therapy and support projects can play an important role in improving self-acceptance.

Acceptance Of Life

Being able to accept your addiction, yourself, and what life throws at you is essential to staying sober. In our seemingly calm and orderly way, life throws constant "keys". Individuals do things that we can do without. Individuals hurt us. We make mistakes. Actually, we can't stand much of life. Either way, we can really control our ability to respond to these opportunities. The moment you accept your life and all the circumstances that come your way, you will experience much greater peace, happiness and support in your recovery. Independence from deepening dependence is a start.

The moment you really work on the most expert method of getting sober and practicing acceptance in your life, the rewards of accumulation will come to you. To most, indoctrinated with alcohol and various substances, it seems so far from the real world. Still trust and confidence. Many have been in your situation, felt the same agony and sorrow, and gone in search of opportunity, inner peace and joy that they have never experienced. You can too.

Tranquility and true serenity are often exceptionally subtle for those dynamically dependent on alcohol. However, it is conceivable and acceptance is the key. Many people drink moderate amounts of alcohol without dangerous results, while for others, just one drink can send them down a risky path. Problem drinking is not only characterized by how often or even how much a person drinks.

All things being equal, it is about the effect of alcohol addiction on a person's life. People who do not like work life, family relationships, finances or emotions at all because of their alcohol consumption may tend to drink excessively. For example, Unwanted or hazardous drinking habits, clinically known as alcohol use disorder, can be serious. In the long term, it can affect the brain and lead to habitual alcohol consumption or addiction.

Mapping a drinking problem is usually difficult but it helps if diagnosed early. Some of the consequences of alcohol addiction can be reversed. Others facing problems with alcohol did not find terms like "drunk" and "alcohol abuse" (or "addict" and "addiction") useless. They may not want to describe themselves as heavy drinkers and may see themselves as someone who struggles with life and abuses alcohol to cope. They may want to reduce their alcohol consumption to a moderate level, rather than stop drinking altogether.

Whether we accept terms like "alcoholic" or "addict," it's important to be careful about how we use them. Accepting that alcohol problems only happen to certain individuals who are "alcoholics" or "addicts" can be a useful way to eliminate potentially very serious alcohol problems in our own lives. Indeed, any of us who drink heavily can cause problems for ourselves and others and may need help to solve those problems, regardless of the words we use to describe ourselves.

In Western culture, alcohol abuse and smoking are two of the most widespread types of addiction. However, they are often considered socially adequate. In the United States, 66% of all adults drink alcohol occasionally. It is estimated that 2 to 10 percent of people over the age of 60 experience side effects of heavy drinking that impair their health and well-being. By definition, these individuals experience the harmful effects of alcohol dependence *(Jinks and Raschko, 1990)*. Assuming smoking is banned, alcohol addiction is the number one drug problem in the United States and in most countries.

Alcohol abuse causes unexpected harm, and the cost of the problem adds billions of dollars to health care in every major country. Men in their 60s still drink nearly as much as they did in their twenties, but fortunately, problem drinking declines in the mid-70s. The prevalence of alcohol dependence and problem drinking is lower in women than in men. The majority of male alcoholics have a strong family alcohol addiction, they start drinking already in everyday life, and they do not become alcoholics little by little, but suddenly and seriously.

CHAPTER 3
THE REASON YOU DRINK

When you feel like this, it's so hard to get the inspiration, clarity, or energy to do anything to move forward. When For a large crowd, a drink or two can be the way to celebrate an event or a proper party. Others may not value alcohol at all; they succeeded without gusto, resentment, or without getting out of control. Assuming you fall into these categories, it can be very difficult to understand why you fall into the drinking problem.

Many people drink when others are drinking around them. In fact, most non-drinkers tend to drink in friendly settings, such as weddings or football matches, where alcohol is considered a real event. Drinking is our general way of life, socially recognized and legal. Peer pressure to drink alcohol can happen at any stage of life. For some people, drinking alcohol is a way of coping with pressure, or if nothing else, they accept it.

Alcohol numbs them to various life problems such as work problems, school problems, relationships, cash, conflicts etc. But amazingly, the problems people try to deal with by drinking can get worse when they drink. In addition, they can contribute to more and more problems. For an alcoholic, an addiction to drinking can turn peer pressure into a cleverly disguised excuse to drink anyway, when they realize they shouldn't because of an increasing rate of trouble.

Alcoholics often admit that they drink to have fun with their friends, which is strangely funny because they sometimes drink alone. Various thought processes associated with drinking alcohol have been analyzed, including drinking to improve friendship, increase strength, get rid of problems, and get high for pleasure or ceremonial reasons. Despite this variability, most studies have focused on two general classifications of inspiration.

The main classification revolves around drinking for pessimistic support, or what Mulford and Miller (1960) called "individual affective intentions". This rationale has been labeled coping drinking and is typically characterized as a tendency to use alcohol to escape, distance, or manage distressing emotions.

The next category revolves around drinking for euphoric feedback, or what Mulford and Miller (1960) called "social influence intentions." This rationale for drinking is labeled "drinking to be polite" and includes drinking to be pleasant, to celebrate social events, and to live with others. It seems reasonable to hypothesize that alcohol consumption is best predicted by people's simultaneous thinking about their drinking thought processes and how their current situation compares to their inspiration.

If another person drinks alcohol primarily to socialize, that person is likely to drink alcohol during social activities; it is during these times that reconciliation takes place between the individual's own thought processes and life circumstances.

In the general consuming population, the amount and frequency of alcohol consumption vary according to the person's circumstances. Going forward, it is necessary to look at the two purposes behind alcohol consumption and how current conditions match those reasons to understand current levels of alcohol consumption. This interaction methodology was analyzed in the General Survey of Alcohol Consumption in Adults. It is estimated that there was a cooperation between drinking motives and ecological conditions.

Even more clearly, people who drink alcohol to cope with stress have been found to have higher alcohol consumption when they are assumed to be under rather than high stress. Similarly, it has been hypothesized that people who drink for social reasons will have higher levels of alcohol consumption, assuming that people in informal communities have high rather than low levels of drinking.

Experts have little idea about the dangers or benefits of moderate alcohol consumption in adults. Almost all lifestyle studies, including diet, exercise, caffeine and alcohol, rely on patient review and honest disclosure of trends over several years. These studies can show that two things can be related, but not necessarily that one causes the other. It is possible that healthy adults engage in more social activities and value moderate alcohol consumption, but alcohol has nothing to do with their recovery.

The potential benefits of alcohol are relatively small and may not have a significant effect on all people. In fact, the latest dietary guidelines clearly state that no one should start consuming or drinking alcohol more often, based on potential medical benefits. For some people, the potential benefits do not outweigh the risks, and staying away from alcohol is the best course of action.

On the other hand, if you happen to be a light to the moderate drinker and are healthy, you can probably continue drinking as long as you do so consciously. What you drink (beer or wine) doesn't seem to matter as much as how you drink. Having 7 drinks on a Saturday night and then not drinking for the rest of the week is nothing compared to one drink a day.

Everything can be very similar from week to week, but the effect on well-being is not. Drinking alcohol at least three or four days a week was inversely associated with the build-up of dead tissue in the heart muscle among members of the Health Care Professionals

Follow-up Study. The amount consumed, less than 10 grams per day or more than 30 grams, did not seem to be as effective as consistency of use. A comparable example was found in Danish men.

Casual Drinking

Occasional drinking is an example of low-risk drinking, which involves consuming small amounts of alcohol from time to time. Careless drinkers, also called social drinkers, consume alcohol regularly, no more than once a week or a few times a month. Regardless of your reasons for drinking, know that there is a difference between occasional drinking and abuse.

Some people cannot drink in moderation and these people are more likely to abuse alcohol. When does casual drinking become alcohol abuse? The short answer is that it's hard to decide. The effect of some (alcoholic) drinks can vary from person to person. In general, what is often considered "safe drinking" has two meanings. The National Institute on Alcohol Abuse and Alcoholism (NIAAA) has its own set of guidelines for what it calls "low-risk" drinking, which sets certain limits on what level of drinking will lead to a later alcohol abuse problem.

That's about three drinks a day and about seven servings a week for women, and about four drinks a day and about 14 drinks a week for men. Abusers consume more alcohol than recommended. However, they do it without thinking, either to manage the pressure or to some extent to the point of complaining about their drinking. An important difference between a heavy drinker and a person with a heavy drinking problem is the ability to reduce drinking or try to stop drinking altogether.

A violent drinker may regret some of the things he did while drunk, but he also has the option of simply cutting down or even

stopping drinking for a while. They don't
have the urge to drink every day, and they
don't struggle with the physical and mental
side effects that alcoholics struggle with.

Occasional drinkers drink regularly. Violent
drunkards complain about their drinking
addiction. In addition, people who drink
because of alcohol dependence not only
complain about drinking, but still cannot
stop or control the urge, and when they think
about it, they often regularly look at the
bottom of their alcohol glass far away and
addiction develops further. It is extremely
important to stop binge drinking because
alcohol addiction can have rare social,
profound and real consequences if left
untreated.

Most alcohol-related problems go
undiagnosed every year and can lead to a
wide spectrum of harmful drinking or
addiction. It is not essential to attend to
consult with your therapist or counselor, and

people are encouraged to self-assess for abuse. There is no quick way out of this. Your body needs time to process alcohol. The morning after a night of heavy drinking, your blood alcohol level will likely be high. You do not have to be healthy or fit to drive.

The legal drink-drive limit indicates the amount of alcohol in your breath, blood or urine. Your body changes as you age. You increased muscle versus fat and decreased body water. This affects how your body processes alcohol. Assuming you drink as much alcohol as you did as an adult, you will feel the effects even more severely.

CHAPTER 4
WHY YOU SHOULD STOP DRINKING

Too much alcohol consumption can cause your blood pressure to ascend in the long run. Following 3-4 weeks of abstaining from alcohol, your blood pressure will begin to decrease. Diminishing your pulse can be vital as it can assist with reducing the risk of medical conditions likely to occur in the future.

As the calories in alcohol can make you put on weight, surrendering alcohol can likewise assist you with lessening your pulse because of the weight you might lose. By this point, on the off chance that you'd recently been drinking six 175ml glasses of alcohol a week, you would have lost 2880 calories in more than three weeks. What's more, in the event that you'd been drinking six pints of larger a week, you would have lost 3240 calories. Alcohol addiction or alcohol abuse and abusive drinking can cause well-being and practical issues that influence the body from head to toe.

The impacts of persistent unreasonable alcohol consumption on different pieces of the endless body frameworks incorporate diminished capacity to learn and recollect, hindered judgment, loss of capacity to reason, poor memory and focus, premature aging of the brain, coronary episode, cardiovascular breakdown, hypertension, sporadic heartbeat, stroke, night blindness, dangerous draining from the throat and stomach, stomach or digestive ulcers, cirrhosis of the liver, greasy liver bringing about unfortunate liver capacity, hepatitis, respiratory sadness prompting demise, interruption of sexual chemicals, fetal irregularities, fetal liquor disorder, pallor (low blood count), expanded diseases due to impaired immunity.

Making a conscious effort to stop consuming alcohol is an extraordinary move toward solid sober living. Whether you've been drinking for a really long time or a couple of months, halting alcohol intake will assist you with confronting life's high points and low points with a more clear psyche and give numerous physical and psychological health benefits. Alcohol is certainly not a solid substance.

Individuals will generally fail to remember that. Without a doubt, there is proof that a couple of drinks can forestall specific sicknesses. Be that as it may, ongoing and hitting the bottle hard is tremendously risky. At the point when somebody drinks exorbitantly, their body is expected to stay at work longer than required to deal with the medication. The liver goes into overdrive to utilize it.

The brain goes haywire as it attempts to align itself. The heart and lungs siphon at sporadic paces. It's not the way that the body is expected to work. Individuals who don't drink, then again, will generally be a lot better. They aren't inclined to alcohol's consequences for the body. Since the body is liberated from handling poisonous synthetics, it can zero in its energy on different things. Subsequently, the psyche and body can work at ideal levels. Moreover, weighty alcohol abuse increases the possibility of dying due to drowning, self-destruction, motor vehicle crashes, and sexually transmitted illnesses.

The actual impacts of alcohol misuse or abuse can incorporate brain damage, chromo-some harm, ongoing bronchitis, expanded defenselessness to contaminations, loss of energy, stomach spasms, and the runs, persistent obstruction, slow and confounded thinking, visual impairment, delirium, mental trips or neurosis, coronary episode, kidney disappointment, punctured nasal septum (the bone and ligament that separates the nasal cavity in two), seizures, stroke, blood clusters to the heart, lung, or mind, a decrease of male and female sex chemicals, easing back the breathing to the mark of unconsciousness or passing, and cellular breakdown in the lungs.

Regardless of whether it obliterates the liver or pancreas, alcohol exhausts the group of B nutrients, vitamin A, and L-ascorbic acid, which are all fundamental for solid physiological working. Sadly, even as liquor "bites up" B nutrients, it impedes the body's capacity to retain these supplements. Exacerbating the situation, consumers frequently substitute alcohol for food, so their admission of B nutrients is low in the first place.

The inadequate intake and trouble utilizing and storing the B vitmins, combined with the body's expanded requirement for them, can set off difficult issues including pallor, muscle, and sensory tissue harm, as well as neurological issues, for example, Korsakoff's condition, which causes transient cognitive decline and trouble learning new data. Likewise, alcohol-related deficiencies of vitamin A can cause night visual deficiency and impeded vision, while too little L-ascorbic acid can debilitate the invulnerable framework, in addition to other things.

Other healthful difficulties of liquor abuse incorporate long-lasting liver harm (or cirrhosis), seizures, diabetes, extreme unhealthiness, and osteoporosis in postmenopausal women. Abstaining from alcohol will emphatically affect your skin because you have better degrees of hydration. As more water will have been consumed instead of squandered, you are probably going to have more hydrated-looking skin, as well as diminished dandruff and dermatitis.

Eliminating alcohol from your eating regimen for a very long time can likewise assist with working on your liver capacity as your liver will begin to shed an overabundance of fat. On the off chance that your liver capacity isn't excessively severely impacted by alcohol, it can recuperate within 4 to 8 weeks. With the liver having an impact in more than 500 fundamental cycles, you likewise allow your body the opportunity of eliminating pollutants, changing over food supplements, and putting away minerals and nutrients.

Excessive alcohol consumption can increase blood pressure in the long term. After 3 weeks of abstinence from alcohol, blood pressure begins to decrease. Reducing your heart rate can be crucial because it can help reduce the risk of diseases that are likely to occur in the future. Because the calories in alcohol can make you gain weight, cutting back on alcohol can also help lower your heart rate because you can lose weight.

If you recently drank six 175ml glasses of alcohol during the week, then you would lose

2880 calories in three weeks. Also, if you drank six liters of alcohol in a week, you would lose 3240 calories. Alcohol dependence or alcohol abuse and drinking can cause well-being and practical problems that affect the body from head to toe.

The effects of chronic excessive alcohol consumption on endless parts of the body include impaired learning and memory, impaired judgment, impaired reasoning, poor memory and concentration, premature aging of the brain, coronary artery disease, cardiovascular disorders, hypertension, irregular heart rhythm, stroke, night blindness, dangerous discharge from the throat and stomach, stomach or gastrointestinal ulcers, liver cirrhosis, fatty liver leading to liver failure, hepatitis, fatal respiratory failure, disruption of sex chemicals, fetal irregularity, fetal drink disorder, pallor (low blood count) and an increase in diseases due to weakened immunity. A conscious effort to stop drinking alcohol is an extraordinary step towards a stable sober life.

Whether you've been drinking for a long time or just a few months, giving up alcohol will help you face life's ups and downs with a clearer mind and bring many benefits to your physical and mental health. Alcohol is not actually a solid substance. People usually don't remember that. There is no doubt that some drinks can prevent some diseases. Be that as it may, hitting the bottle constantly and hard is extremely risky. If someone drinks too much, their body is expected to stay working longer than it takes to process the drug.

The liver goes into overdrive to utilize it. The brain messes up trying to align itself. The heart and lungs beat randomly. This is not how the body is supposed to work. People who don't drink are usually much better. They are not prone to the effects of alcohol on the body. As the body is freed from processing toxic synthetic substances, it can revitalize itself in a variety of ways. Then, the mind and body can function at an ideal level. In addition, heavy alcohol abuse increases the chance of dying from drowning, self-harm, motor vehicle accidents, and sexually transmitted diseases.

Actual effects of alcohol abuse can include brain damage, chromosomal damage, permanent bronchitis, increased defenses against pollution, loss of energy, stomach cramps and running, persistent congestion, slow and confused thinking, visual impairment, delirium, mental disorders or neurosis, coronary disease episodes, kidney failure, tear in the nasal septum (the bone and ligament that divides the nasal cavity in half), seizures, stroke, blood clots in the heart, lungs or mind, male and female sex chemicals, easy breathing, loss of consciousness or fainting, and cell rupture in the lungs.

Whether it destroys the liver or the pancreas, alcohol depletes the B nutrients, vitamin A and L-ascorbic acid, all of which are essential for sound physiological function.

Unfortunately, while alcohol "bites" the B nutrients, it interferes with the body's ability to store these extra nutrients. The situation is made worse by the fact that consumers often trade food for alcohol, so the absorption of B nutrients is low in the first place. Inadequate intake of B vitamins and difficulty using and storing them, as well as the body's increased need for them, can cause serious problems such as pallor, damage to muscle and sensory tissues, and neurological problems such as Korsakoff's condition can cause temporary problems. Cognitive impairment and difficulty learning new information.

Likewise, alcohol-related vitamin A deficiencies can cause a lack of night vision and impaired vision, while too little L-ascorbic acid can weaken the invulnerable frame, among other things. Other health problems associated with alcohol abuse include long-term liver damage (or cirrhosis), seizures, diabetes, extreme malaise, and osteoporosis in postmenopausal women. Abstaining from alcohol will greatly affect your skin as you will have better hydration levels.

Because more water has been used instead of wasted water, your skin is likely to look more hydrated and less prone to dandruff and breakouts. Cutting alcohol out of your diet for a very long time can also help improve your liver capacity as your liver begins to break down excess fat. If alcohol does not affect the liver too severely, it can recover in 8 weeks.

Because the liver affects more than 500 basic cycles, you give your body a chance to eliminate impurities, remove supplements, and release minerals and nutrients. Most people who don't drink too much alcohol have no problem not drinking anything else after a few drinks. However, occasional heavy drinking can cause a hangover due to the build-up of the harmful metabolite acetylaldehyde. It causes hangovers, sweating, palpitations, and general nausea/excessiveness with the headache.

If you are not particularly prone to alcohol or do not drink regularly, these side effects should disappear in at least a day or two. People who are truly dependent on alcohol may experience long-term withdrawal symptoms. These can range from less than overwhelming problems (such as sweating, increased blood pressure, heart rate, and anxiety) to psychosis, delirium, seizures, and death.

CONCLUSION

Recovery is indeed a long-term cycle that changes the actions of the recovering person emphatically every day, if not from moment to moment. Recovery often changes a person's goals, expectations, behavior and even character. Thus, these changes can also vary from person to person. In fact, people should feel much better within the first few weeks of quitting. Alcohol does not stay long in the body.

In fact, even long-distance drinkers can detox in a week or two. If they eat healthy and exercise, they should feel better in no time. But drinking also has an emotional impact and profound side effects. If a heavy drinker has a co-occurring disorder, such as anxiety, the condition will continue after they stop drinking. Be that as it may, abstinence from alcohol can help them achieve stability. If they turn to an expert for help and focus on moderation, their psychological state should reach the next level. The benefits of alcohol rehabilitation are not just physical. It can also have financial benefits.

All things considered, as anyone who drinks knows, the price of alcohol can add up. A couple of beers or a bottle of wine only cost a few dollars. In any case, if someone drinks every day or even every week, the costs add up after a while. Bad money choices are often associated with drinking. When a legal problem like a DUI arises, it costs a lot. There are many reasons why you should stop drinking alcohol. For some people, it's a lifestyle change - say goodbye to hangovers, get better rest, lose a decent amount of weight and have more energy.

It could even be a challenge to another person or a fundraiser for a noble cause. For others, stopping drinking may be essential for clinical reasons. Perhaps due to alcohol-related medical conditions such as liver disease, or the fact that they are taking medications that react strongly with alcohol. Whatever the explanation, fortunately, anyone can stop alcoholism or drinking. Also, if you're considering cutting alcohol out of your life, you're not alone.